Plantar Fasciitis:

Surprisingly sensible instructions for plantar fasciitis sufferers

By

Zoé Rios

Contents

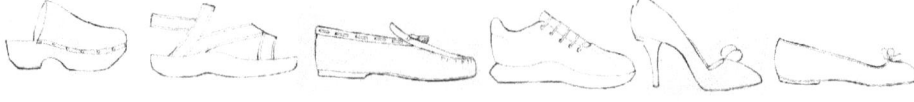

1. What causes Plantar Fasciitis?

Some people call plantar fasciitis an overuse injury. I prefer to see it more as an underuse problem. It is the result of continued use of a certain type of shoe or orthotic that reduces the amount of motion needed for walking. With less day-to-day motion of certain areas of the foot, the fascia slowly tightens and becomes vulnerable to tears and irritation. The same restricted motion can also cause a weakening of muscles in the feet in turn increasing the pressure on the fascia when not supported by the shoe or orthotic.

Shoes that cause plantar fasciitis by reducing motion are often seen as supportive or comfort shoes. They are comfortable because your foot has to do less work. The shoe supports your foot as high tech rubber soles and insoles propel you forward and surround your foot softly and effectively protecting your foot from the ground.

Plantar fasciitis can also become a problem after wearing orthotics, often prescribed to heal an injury which could be anything from a broken or fractured bone to a pulled tendon or trapped nerve.

Orthotics are a very effective way of immobilizing the foot in order to allow healing, however whenever you immobilize, there will always be loss in muscle tone and tightening of tissue including fascia.

It is important to remember that your feet are made up of bones, nerves, muscles, tendons and fascia and just like the rest of your body, they require proper movement to remain healthy. After healing from a broken arm you would expect to need to carefully stretch and strengthen when the cast comes off. You should expect to do the same for your feet.

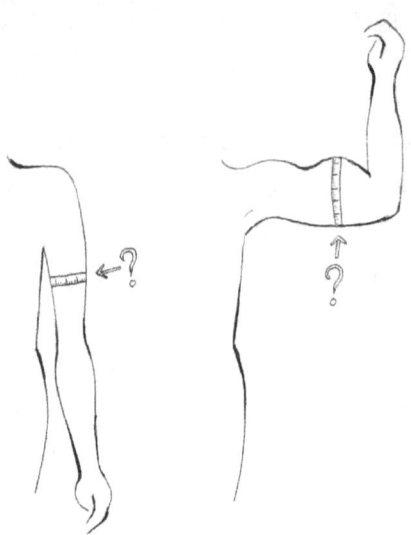

Orthotics and arch supports not only make motion not required but they actually prevent the muscles in the foot from working.

When a muscle contracts it changes shape and requires a different space. If the area under the arch is filled in, the plantar muscle cannot contract. Additionally the skin under the arch is very sensitive, if the arch area is filled in but the shoe does not recreate the momentum necessary, the skin under the arch will become sore very quickly.

When A to B shortens, H to B lengthens, if A to B cannot shorten the distance to H cannot change either. This is why filling in the arch area causes the top-line of certain shoes to slip.

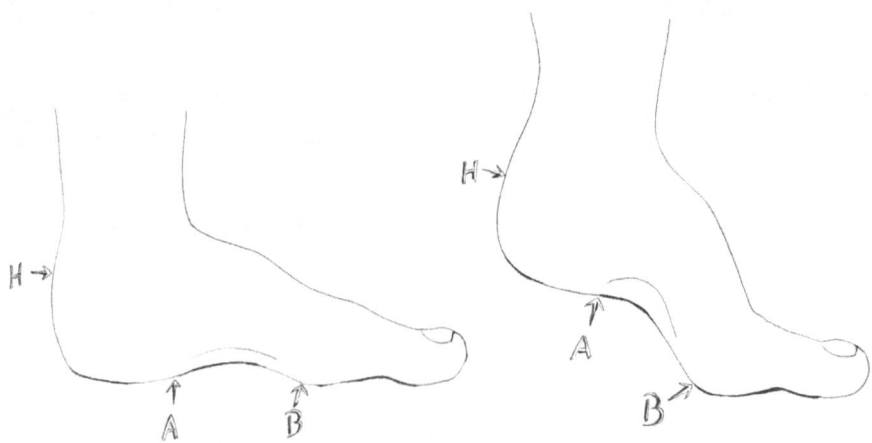

Problem

The problem that most people have and possibly the reason you are reading this book is that the cure for plantar fasciitis is also the cause. Frustrated sufferers find themselves in a painful cycle of an ever worsening catch 22 that they don't know how to fix, and the pain always comes back with vengeance.

Solution

After years of asking sufferers to follow a regime of careful exercise and stretching, I have established a formula of rehabilitation that most people find easy to follow and if followed correctly have consistently successful results.

It is important to recognize that this is a treatment plan for plantar fasciitis and pain resulting from tight fascia. If your pain is in a very specific area you should ask your MD to check that it is not a stress fracture or other ailment. Your MD can prescribe an orthotic for heeling. The treatment plan outlined in this book can be started when the injury has healed and you are ready for rehabilitation to begin.

It is common for people to assume that exercise for your feet should happen at the same time as exercise for the rest of your body, however trying to do this often leads people to either sacrifice their regular workout miss their walk or run with friends and gain weight. Or, push their feet too far to fast and incur a setback. Instead, I encourage people especially in the beginning but possibly long term to use whatever shoe and orthotic combination they need in order to get their normal exercise done and use the rest of the day to exercise their feet. Once general foot health is back you will have the option to go one stage further and aim for optimum foot strength.

2. The Basic Plan

1. Change shoes.

The most important part of this plan requires you to wear at least two different types of shoes each day. If you go to work all day you must take a second pair and change shoes during the day. If, your day includes a workout, you must use a separate pair of shoes for your workout and not wear your workout shoes for anything other than working out.

All shoes are both good and bad. Different types of shoes use different muscles and have different pressure points. They all cause injuries in different ways if worn for too long or for the wrong activity. They all protect in different ways and have different benefits.

In the next chapter I will talk more about shoe styles and how they effect your feet giving you an overview that will help you understand what to wear and when.

2. Get moving.

Establish an exercise and stretching routine for your feet that can be done at any time of the day. Chapters 4 & 5 will give you some ideas to get started, the exercises are simple and as you grow to understand the goal you may find that local yoga instructors and physical therapists are a great resource for new exercises that add variety to your routine.

3. Shoe styles and how they effect your feet.

There are pros and cons with all shoes however, wearing the same type of shoe all day every day puts you at risk for an over use injury from that particular style. Importantly, it also puts you at risk for side effects of under use of certain muscles due to slightly restricted movement.

It can also be confusing as to which shoe does what. The most important design criteria that dictate the way the shoe works are not always obvious to the untrained eye leading people to think they are wearing a different style shoe when actually their shoe choices are all creating the same problem.

Here I have divided the basic shoe styles into categories, detailing specific characteristics that dictate which category a shoe belongs in. Although there may be other differences that could make you wonder why the shoes belong in the same category, the categories are divided specifically for the way they interact with your foot.

When a shoe is made, it is 'lasted', pulled tight over a last or form in the shape of a foot. The shape of the last and way in which the fabric or leather is pulled onto the last dictates how the shoe will act on the foot. The last is chosen by the designer to perform best for certain activities and with certain materials, which is why one is not necessarily better than the other. In recent years fashions have made popular the use of an athletic style construction for alternate uses, making comfort shoes popular to wear more often.

One of the easiest ways to exercise your feet is to simply change shoes to a different style. Resting and exercising a different set of muscles in your feet while walking, standing and going about your daily life.

The reason for changing your shoes in the middle of the day rather than alternating a whole day at a time is that for most people their feet will become too tired and they will become overly sore in the opposing style shoes that they are not used to.

To begin with you may need to switch shoes even more frequently.

Group 1.

Hard soled protective.

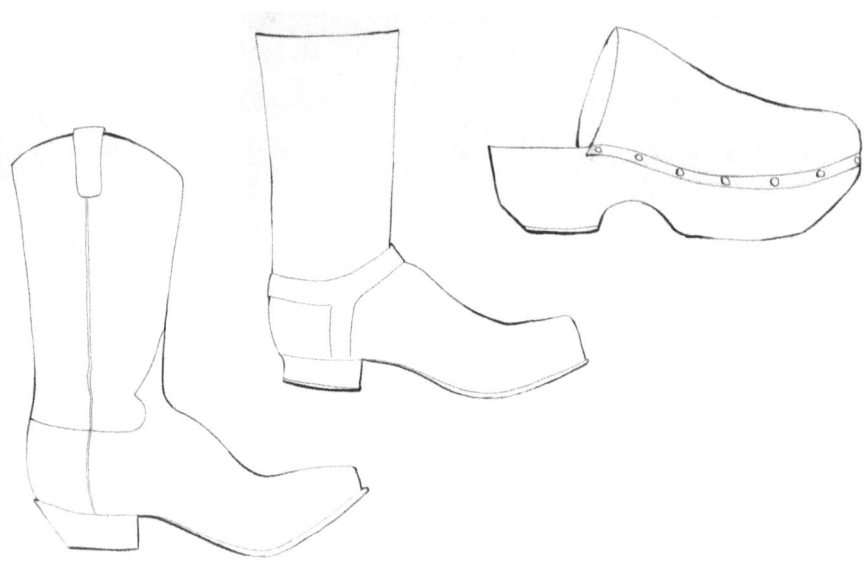

These include protective footwear with a relatively stiff sole, wooden clogs, cowboy boots and biker boots. The heels and toes curve up causing a rocker action as you move forward compensating for the stiffness. The pressure point where the shoe or boot holds on is almost at the crease in the ankle, above the navicular (the lumpy bone on the top that moves upwards when the arch is engaged). The arch can still move and there is a slight movement of the heel in the boot as you step forward.

The slight movement in the heel means that orthotics slip out of place easily, most people do not chose to wear them with this type of shoe.

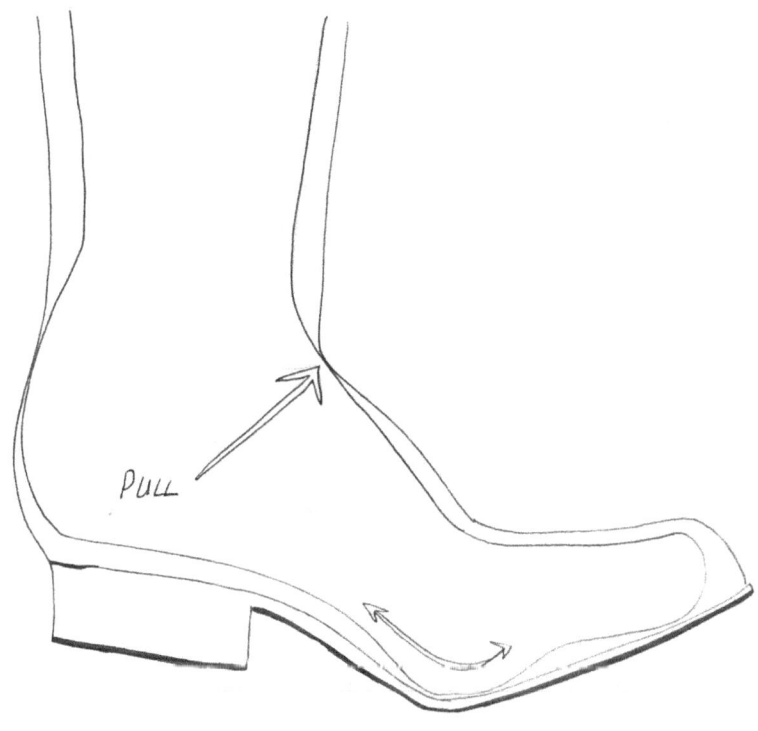

PULL

When you get a new pair of leather boots they may slip a little at the heel. This stops when the sole has settled into the wearers natural mid-stride position. A properly fitting boot rocks forward in perfect timing with the lifting of the arch.

Group 2.

Cushioned.

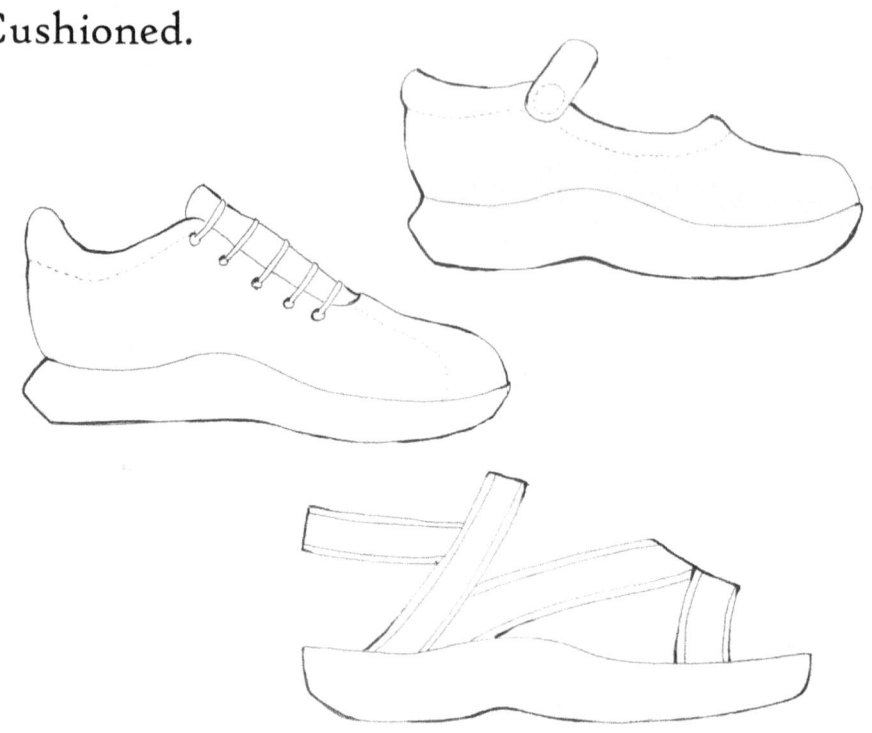

These include all cushioned athletic shoes, all cushioned comfort shoes, thick contoured sandals, basically anything with a cushioned sole.

The cushioning while delaying the ground response also makes it un-necessary.

The shoe also uses advanced cushioning materials to propel the wearer forward. The lacing or strap system is designed to hold the foot as firmly in place as it can without restricting blood flow.

This type of shoe is a good choice for wearing with orthotics as it is designed to work without propulsion from the arches.

This shoe will protect the wearer from over exertion in the foot but also poses the highest risk of weakening of muscle tone and stiffness from reduced motion.

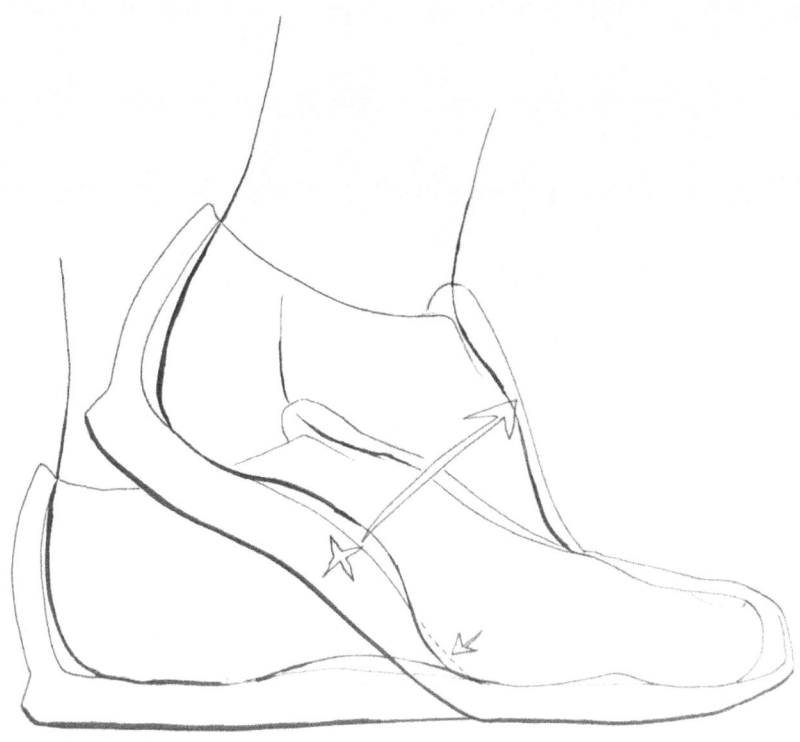

The pitch and spring of the sole mean that less motion is required from the foot in order to move forward comfortably. If there is still some change in shape of the foot, it is absorbed with interior cushioning. The interior cushioning makes room for the ball joint preventing the extra ball joint volume, against the wide stabilizing sole, from shoving the foot forward when flexed. Cushioning creates instability, the extra width in the sole compensates recreating stability.

Well designed athletic shoes use all of these components in balance to create an enhanced forward propulsion.

A poorly fitting or poorly designed shoe can cause tightness in the hips or friction injuries (blisters).

Group 3.

Thin and flexible.

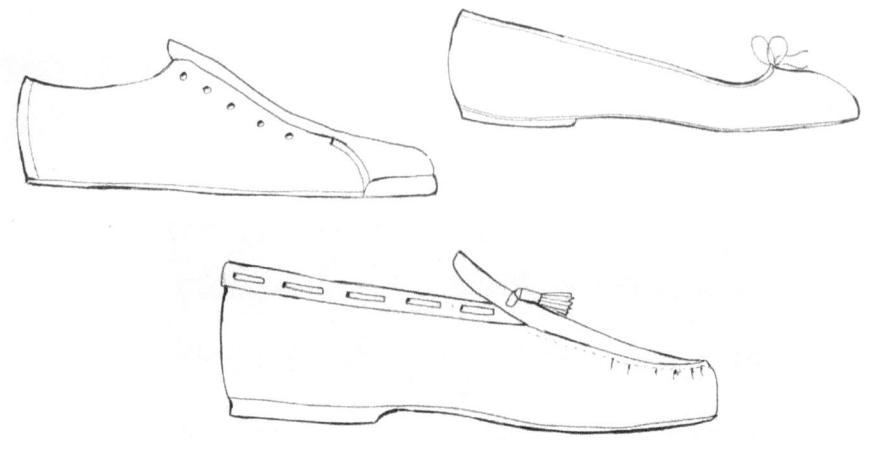

This group includes shoes with less than 1/4 inch of cushioning and do not have a padded collar around the top of the heel.

Old style plimsoles, ballet flats, deck shoes, driving shoes and some men's dress shoes all come in this category however sometimes cushioned shoes are designed to look like these styles. If there is extra padding, they must go in group 2.

These shoes allow full motion in the arches. When you step forward the arch lifts, changing the angle of the heel which lengthens the distance from the ball joint to the back of the top line. Even lace up versions should have enough flexibility to allow proper movement in the arch.

People who have difficulty finding the correct fit for their feet often have difficulty holding some of these styles on, clenching their toes and being unable to walk with a relaxed foot prevents the top line from functioning properly making the problem worse. A lace-up or maryjane is the best choice for these people.

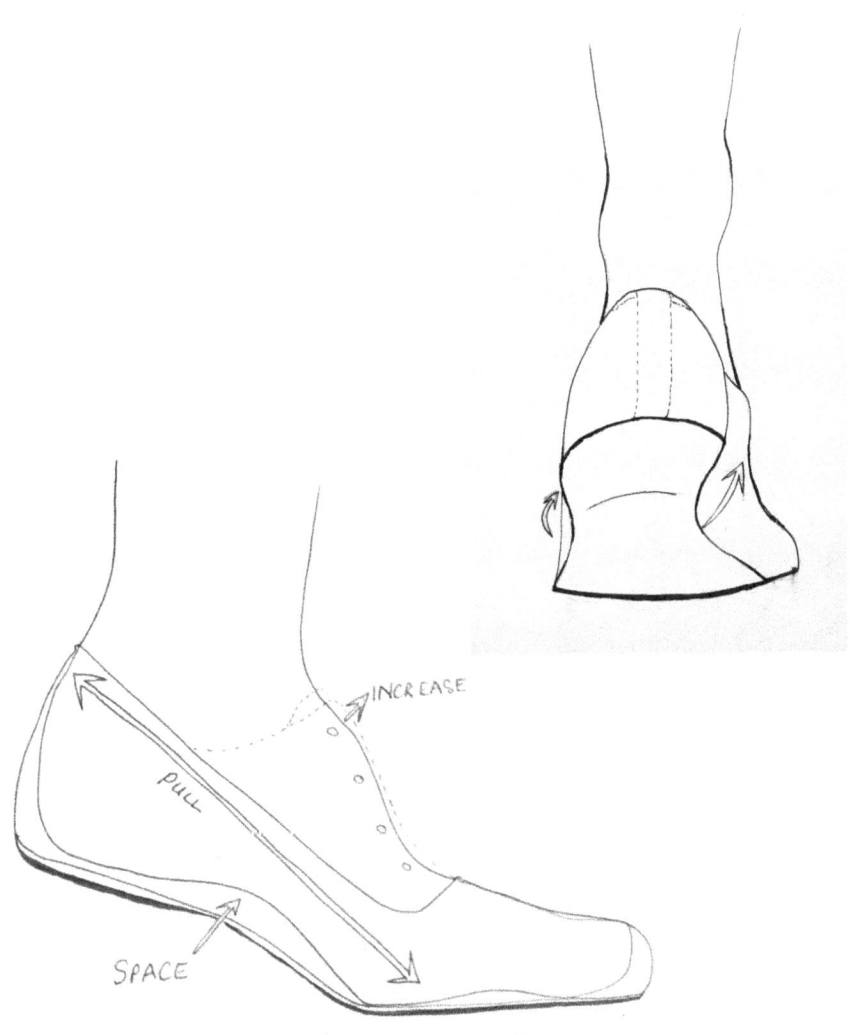

The arch increase is able to happen properly when the leather or fabric under the arch area is soft enough to move. That's why 'old fashioned' shoes have a narrow sole under the instep or 'waist'. The filling in of the arch area for 'arch support' prevents the fabric from moving upwards and acts like a tie-down for the arch.

Group 4.

Other.

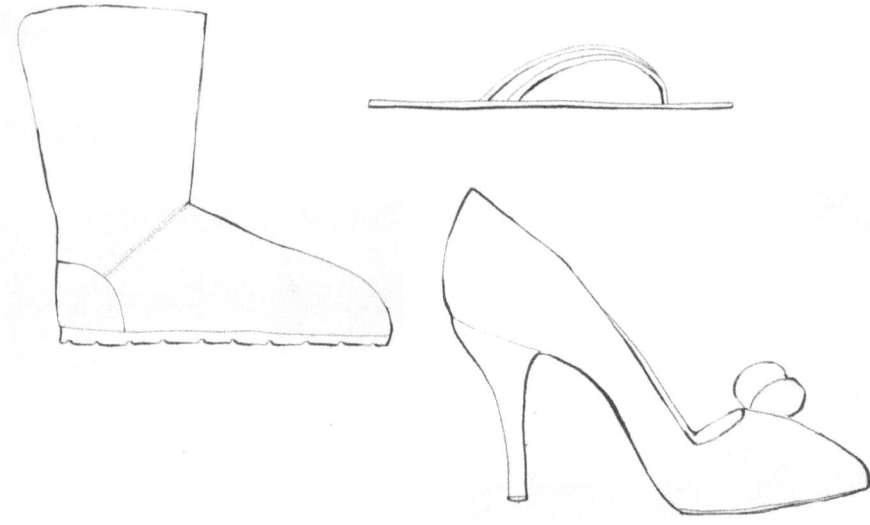

This group includes a great variety, most of which you would never dream of wearing for more than a couple of hours.

Aside from high heels, these types of shoes are not strapped tightly to your foot, if you try to walk too far in them, you could suffer discomfort from trying to hold them on, or having to pick your feet up more carefully to prevent them from dragging.

The injuries that high heels cause are blisters, calluses and aching ball joints. Most people take their shoes of when these ailments become a problem, saving themselves from a more long term injury.

When it comes to footwear, variety causes short bursts of using apposing muscles. You should be able to have fun and wear what you want **as long as you change shoes when your feet hurt.**

How to begin

If you take your shoes off and launch immediately into a new foot strengthening regime, the sudden increase in movement will likely make the small tears in the fascia that are already bothering you, much worse. The first tears may have happened from simply taking one little step out of bed after a night of rest. Your planter muscles were not quite strong enough to support your arch high enough against your body weight to prevent the tightened fascia from stretching just a little past its capacity.

If your plantar fasciitis is particularly bad you will need to find a shoe or boot from group 1. that you can tolerate and that increases the arch motion just a little, start by wearing for only short periods of time. Many of my customers have had success with a good pair of leather cowboy boots. Pay attention to how your feet feel and switch back to your old orthotics and/or comfort shoes when your feet are tired.

Next try including shoes from groups 3 & 4.

The goal is to work up to wearing 2 pairs of shoes a day, alternating from each of the four groups.

Gaining weight without gaining the corresponding foot strength needed to support the weight will cause set-backs and possible additional injuries. I recommend that you continue to use whatever orthotics and advanced footwear you need in order to do your normal workout. You should consider your foot strengthening program as something that you do separately, especially at first but possibly all the time.

Wear shoes designed for the activity you are doing, running shoes for running, flip flops for the beach etc. When you finish your workout you should change shoes and not wear your exercise shoes when you are not exercising.

You can begin a foot stretching regime from the beginning and once you are comfortably wearing shoes from at least three groups you can start adding in more exercises.

4. Stretching

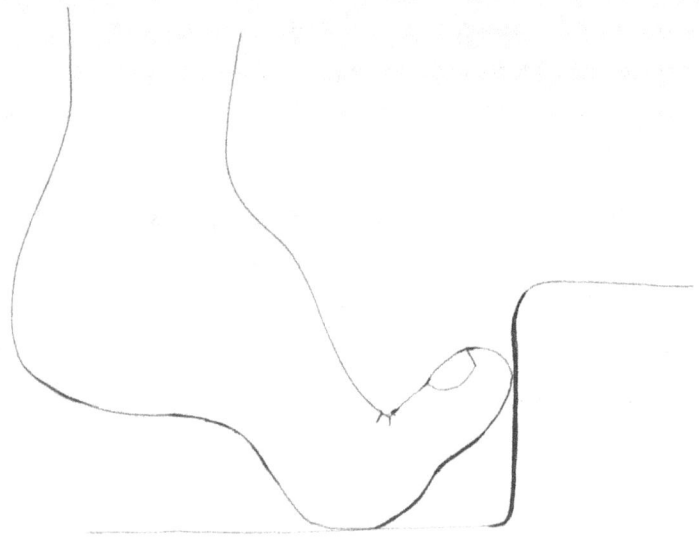

Stretching should be done slowly and feel good.

Tendons are like ropes and if you've ever found a tendon while slicing through a piece of meat you will realize it's probably not going to stretch. Muscles do stretch though and in this case the goal is to gently stretch the plantar muscle that runs along the bottom of your foot. The best way to do this is to gently pull your big toe towards your shin. Another way is to press your big toe up against a firm surface like a curb or step and push your leg forward as if to take a step, both with your knee straight and flexed. You should be able to experience a nice stretch all the way from your toe to the top of your calf at the same time.

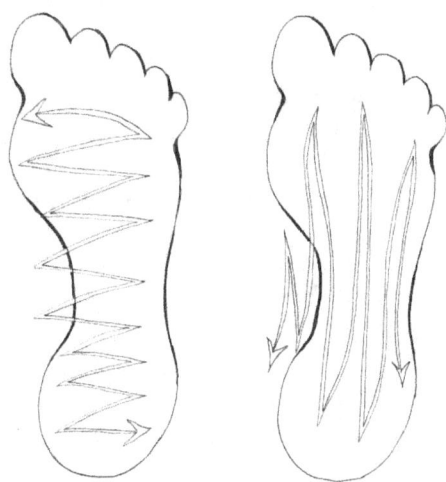

You should also roll a small ball under your feet.

You can buy a special foot stretching ball, which I'm sure will work well. Rubber bouncy balls that you can buy at any discount store also work well and you can find one that fits your foot, large enough to reach all the way into your arch and yet small enough to feel good.

Many of my customers who have children confess to finding a free one in the back of the sofa although investing 50 cents on one that feels just right is well worth the investment.

Roll the ball gently in the pattern you see above, it should feel good.

You should do both stretches every day and there is no harm in stretching more if you want to.

Massage therapists and trainers very often have different and interesting stretches, you should add in other stretches in addition to these but not replace.

Stretching makes a big difference but very slowly. People often ask me how long it takes to stretch out your feet after they have become stiff. The answer is that everyone is different. How long would it take you to learn how to do the splits?

5. Exercise

- Switching shoes, walking and going about your day to day life in a variety of footwear is the first and most important exercise.

Once you have made some progress and you are able to tolerate walking around your house with bare feet you may begin extra foot exercises to speed up your road to fully fit feet.

- Picking small objects and pencils up with your toes, wiggling your toes and rotating your feet in circles while your toes are relaxed. The goal is to get your circulation moving and increase the blood flow throughout your foot all the way to the tips of your toes.

- Heel raises, should be started when you are ready and if your weight is in the healthy range. At first you should hold onto a firm countertop or the back of a chair, as your feet get stronger you can begin to let go, adding balance into the challenge.

When this becomes easy you can work your way up to assisted then unassisted single foot raises.

You should pay close attention to how your feet feel, and stop when your feet are tired.

In order to make progress strengthening any muscle group, you have to learn to work hard enough to make the muscle group tired un-yet learn to stop before injury. Most people learn how to distinguish this difference while lifting weights in the gym. The same principle applies to your feet, work hard but increase slowly.

There are many physical therapists and trainers who recommend all kinds of exercises that I have not mentioned. Yoga instructors are also a great resource for foot exercises. Seeking further tips from well qualified professionals will add variety to your routine, I highly recommend you research resources in your area.

6. Maintenance

Once you have returned to normal foot health you may be able to resume more normal shoe wearing habits and perhaps go the whole day in one pair of shoes without disappearing to your car for the necessary foot wardrobe change, but only if you continue at least part of the regimen. Wear one pair all day, then exercise and stretch, or, change shoes and not worry about special exercises. After recovery, moderation should be possible without slipping back to your old ways.

Importantly, do not wear athletic shoes all day.

It is important to remember that loss of flexibility and mobility is a natural consequence of getting older. Nobody gets younger, and without continued effort to stay in motion, tightening fascia followed by plantar fasciitis can always return. Weight gain is also one of the biggest reasons for deteriorating foot health. If you gain a few pounds while wearing a variety of shoe styles and frequently walking in a safe area with bare feet your feet will gain strength simultaneously. If you gain weight while wearing very supportive shoes, you will not gain the necessary strength and put yourself at risk of injury.

It is important to remember that this program is for rehabilitation and not a cure for all injuries. You may at some point experience a different injury which should be treated with the use of a custom orthotic. You will need to heal properly then start this program again from the beginning.

7. Running

Running can be a wonderful way to stay slim, fit and happy, visit with friends and get outside. Modern cushioned running shoes make this great lifestyle choice available to many who perhaps would otherwise not have the strength. It is important to remember though that if you are using a cushioned shoe, your feet are not experiencing the same level of activity as the rest of your body.

There are two reasons cushioned running shoes can be bad. The first is that if you wear them all day, you will not be exercising your feet properly and muscle depletion can cause all the problems we've just discussed. The solution to this is to simply not wear your running shoes for anything other than running and to think about exercising your feet separately, at a different time of the day.

The second problem from cushioned running shoes is that they can increase impact further up your body, this is particularly serious if you do not have good form, over striding and landing on a straight leg causes many injuries. If you are able to land on a bent knee with every stride, you may experience little consequence to the shoes and again proper stretching and exercise at another time of the day may be all you need to do for optimum health.

Additionally, if you do decide to take up minimal shoe running there is no reason to think that you must never don a specialized pair of shoes to maximize your performance when you want to. You may find it difficult to go back, but you cannot undo your strength in one day.

Some of the nay-sayers of minimal shoes have published studies on how much extra energy you can save with cushioned shoes. I agree with them, except I have difficulty understanding why this is a problem consuming more calories while transitioning is not hard for most people. You are increasing strength in more small muscles which I think most trainers agree is good. I also think there could be other important metabolic benefits. I am only seeing the beginning of a few studies on this topic, it'll be interesting to see what conclusions people come to about this in the future.

8. Minimal Shoe Running

Running in minimal shoes with proper form will reduce the impact on your knees, hips and back. Cushioning prevents your body from reacting to the ground. When your body has enough strength to protect it's self properly with flexed muscles the result is astonishingly effective. The moment the nerves in your feet feel the hard surface they send messages that cause the body to respond. The thicker the shoe the more time it takes for the body to respond. Also when your foot feels softness it tells your knees to brace and stabilize which is the opposite to what you want if you've just landed your foot on a cement sidewalk. Socks are soft but they also absorb moisture and prevent friction in a minimal shoe. The best compromise I've found thus far is thin cotton socks in the summer and thin wool socks in the winter.

Shoes add stiffness or resistance to the initial lifting of your heel of the ground, which is why they have a pitch or raised heel. A minimal shoe without cushioning gives no protection to your heel, making it necessary to eliminate the pitch to zero. With zero pitch the stiffness can cause injury to your Achilles tendon. The best option here is to chose the most flexible shoe available.

The second important consideration is that the navicular (bone on top of your foot at the arch) must be able to move up and outwards in order for your arch to be able to do its job properly. Shoes that do not have a padded top line collar and are designed to hold on at the heel are best for this arch motion. Lace your shoes with your heel raised and ball flexed to ensure you leave enough room.

The third and possibly the most important consideration is foot strength and how to obtain strong enough feet to protect the rest of your body. Injury to your knees only happens if you land on a knee that is not bent. This in the running world is known as over striding. Speed must come from toe push-off which requires strength. A good way to find out if you have enough foot strength to run, is to try skipping, step-hop-step-hop etc. If you are strong enough to skip and make it well of the ground you should be able to run.

A good way to prepare is doing single foot heel raises. At first you should run very slowly and practice getting the proper distance of the ground instead of worrying about distance travelled and learn to listen to your body. If your feet begin to feel sore, walk, if your calves become sore, walk, if your toes begin to hurt, walk.

When you first begin running with minimal shoes and your feet aren't really strong enough you might feel like your doing more of a hobble or a fast walk.

It might feel like you are running on the outside of your feet.

You will need to find the 'sweet' spot when you land. In order to do this you must relax your feet and keep your shoulders back.

The first part of your foot to touch the ground should be the padded bit behind the little toe, prior to where it flexes. You will next find out that the motion in your lateral arch may be so small that you might never have noticed using it before, however it provides just enough distance for your foot to provide precise protection from a hard surface.

Until you have developed proper muscle memory you will need to keep reminding yourself of key things.

- Relax feet

- Shoulders back

- Head up

- Knees bent, don't over stride

- Watch where you tread!

Some advice that Christopher Mc Dougal gives in his book *Born to Run,* is to, "run like a bird". This is good thought, although after three or four years of running with correct form your feet may become so much stronger that you begin to notice a much more fluid motion, you will feel less like a goose on Christmas morning and more like your body was meant to do this.

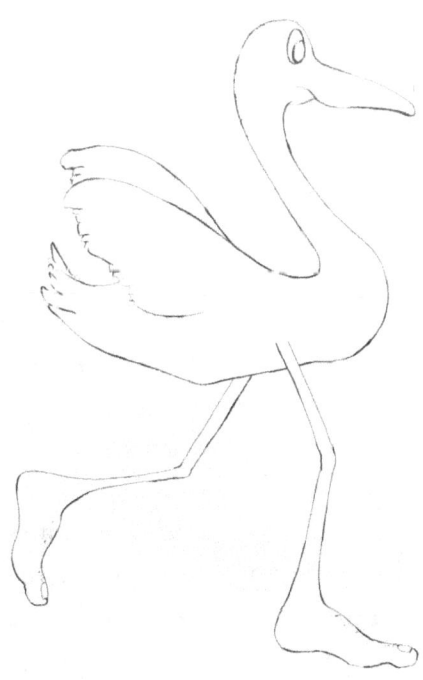

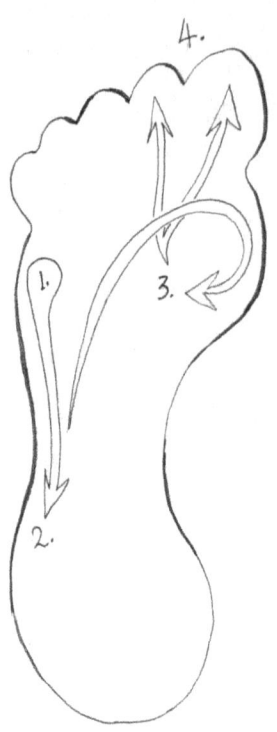

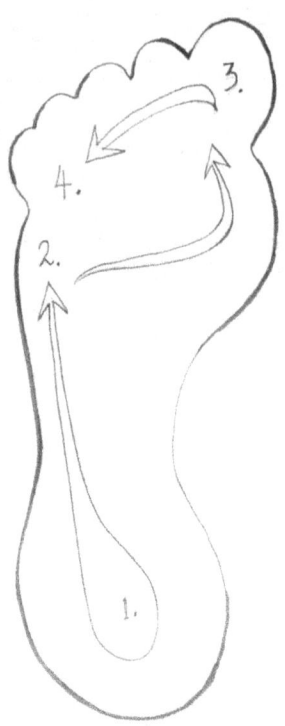

Walking

1. The fat pad touching down begins to determine the body's response, softening for a hard surface or bracing for stability.

1-2 Lateral arch flexes to reduce impact

2-4 The transverse & medial arch rotates down, pushing the ball to the ground allowing the foot to roll onto the big toe

3-4 As the body weight passes over, the arch draws up increasing angle of the ball joint adds pressure to the toes to complete push off.

Running & Skipping

1. Relaxed foot touches the ground here.

1-2 Lateral arch flexes down for initial impact protection

2-3 Transverse arch flexes down to engage ball joint and initiate raising of the medial arch for lift off.

3-4 Medial arch raises and engages the downward pressure of the toes for propulsion

9. Who knows what and why.

There are some shoe companies with a long history of good design knowledge. It is important to research the company when deciding who's design to trust your feet to though.

In the beginning of my learning experience, I assumed that shoes and lasts were designed by someone who knew how to make shoes and exactly how that shoe would effect your body. Once becoming qualified as a pedorthist, I was shocked to realize that the founding designers of a few big shoe companies, where qualified only as a pedorthist with no last or shoe making experience. Many times it is a design engineer with a qualification in computer design that makes critical decisions that dictate how the shoe effects your health. Unscrupulous marketing encouraging the miss-use of sport or orthopedic shoes preventively is rampant.

The shoe industry has gone through some profound changes that the education system has only recently begun to catch up to. Despite school based study, much of my useful knowledge came from traditional boot and shoemakers who themselves learnt from other boot and shoemakers. I would encourage you to chose your advisors diligently and pick professionals carefully. Here's a brief summery of common practitioners:

- Orthopedic MD - The only person you should trust to judge if you should make changes to your shoes that could alter the angle of your joints.

- Orthetist - Fabricates orthopedic devises prescribed by the MD knows about shoes from group 2.

- Pedorthist- Fabricates orthopedic devises from the knee or ankle down, prescribed by the MD, also has extensive knowledge about shoes in group 2.

- Certified shoe fitter- Has mostly studied about shoes in group 2. May claim to be able to analyze gait however has no training in how modifications to the footwear could effect the rest of the kinetic chain. You should only take advise on fit!

If anyone claims you pronate or supinate too much or too little, you should understand that your foot may be compensating for problems with knees, hips or back. Always check with the MD before altering anything.

People often assume that support in a shoe means arch support and to all the people in the previous list who have only studied shoes in group 2, this is where they may think it is.

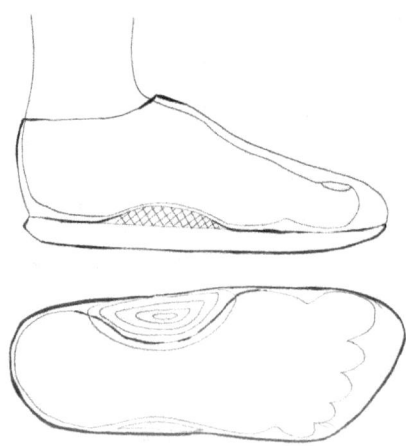

Shoemakers who are looking beyond shoes that restrict arch movement think that shoe support is in the structure of the shoe or boot that prevents the surface that you are standing on from becoming concave. A poorly made or designed shoe can have support added. In which case it is added just behind the ball joint in the center of the foot. That is why a well made leather soled or in-soled shoe maintains good support for longer than a soft shoe subject to compression.

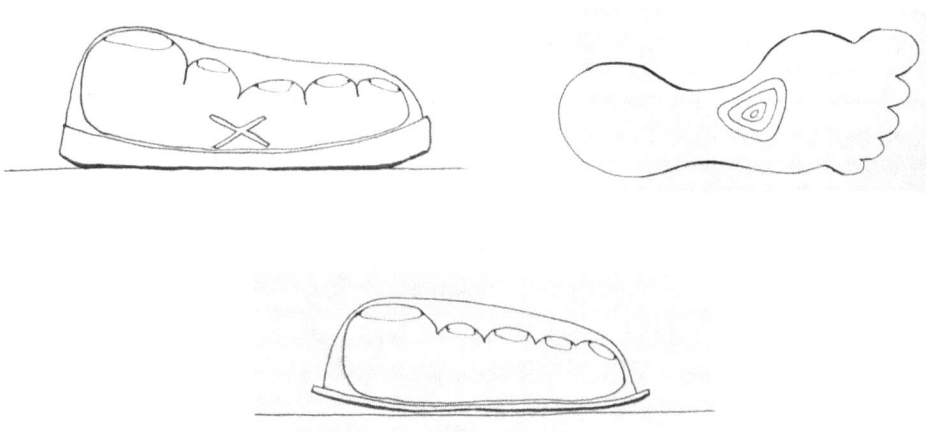

Recently there has been a surge of people learning how to make traditional shoes by hand combined with a new crop of excellent shoe and bootmaking schools.

I would recommend that if you have the opportunity to invest in good handmade shoes they are likely to serve you well. Very few shoe and bootmakers study pedorthics nor do they need to. Most do not study shoes in group 2. They become experts in either one or two of the other groups of shoes. Importantly they quickly become experts in fit, and the quality of the materials that they use often lends itself to better foot health and longer lasting support.

10. My Story, How I know what I know

Everybody asks, but I'm not entirely sure who really wants to know the whole story, for this reason it seems like a good idea to put it in writing, that way you can simply stop reading when you've heard enough about me. In fact if you stop right here, you'll know all you need to know, the rest is just for curiosity. If anyone asks if you read the whole book, the answer if you got this far is yes.

Despite many strange adventures, I've never really thought of myself as a risk-taker. For instance, if I have a dollar, I'd rather save it and earn .2% interest than I would buy a lottery ticket. Risk takers might not consider all the options properly, I seem to just have different priorities in the things I consider most important.

I left the beginnings of a promising career in the fashion industry in London in my early twenties, for a 'year out' with a poorly planned ending. My career did not get back on track for multiple years, but when it did I found it important not to waste the wisdom gained from the years of life experiences I'd stumbled through.

In the beginning I skied a lot. I worked for a British tour company, took care of vacationing skiers and skied. I skied so much that I needed to increase the challenge and so decided to forgo my downhill skis for early generation tele-mark, free-heeling leather boots and skinny skis. After an exhausting third winter I began to understand the relationship of movement and stability or balance and motion.

Next I landed a job as a flight attendant, on a whim, in response to a full page advertisement. Flying enabled me to indulge in abundant people watching and the joy of working with a fantastically diverse group of people.

As part of my uniform, I was required to wear black leather pumps. My English upbringing instilled in me a discomfort in changing shoes in public, so despite all my American colleagues switching between two different pairs, I invested in a good leather pair imported from a well-established Italian designer and wore them all day every day.

My feet swelled up from time to time from the cabin pressure changes and poor nutritional options. Each new pair gave me blisters at the beginning before becoming comfortable and I kicked them of the moment I arrived home or at the hotel. Everyone else would opt for a higher heel and carry a second pair of flats in their bag which they switched into on every flight. We were on our feet fourteen hours a day and charged from plane to plane at a frantic pace frequently bursting into an inter-terminal run. I worked with different crews almost every month and in almost ten years never met anyone who had plantar fasciitis.

I did have one foot injury. Rapidly descending in the back galley of an old style plane with horribly outdated horizontal flap cabinets I gave the cabinet one last kick with the ball of my foot to prevent my exit from becoming blocked with flying food carriers. It was a little painful for a few days, I ignored it. Three or four weeks later a small painful callus appeared in the same spot.

I went to a reputable podiatrist who explained I had a bone spur, a small chip that I realized must have come from the dispute with the uncompliant cabinet. He cast me for a functional, dress orthotic which I wore in my shoes for the next couple of months after which I appeared to be completely better. Despite the fact that he gave me no instruction to discontinue use, they caused my shoes to not hold on properly and slip at the heel so with my injury healed I took them out. This experience proved to be most useful in later years, having experienced first-hand the proper use of orthotics.

Controversially, one of my greatest priorities while making important life decisions is not to miss out on a great opportunity or adventure. This led me to be married to a tall black haired Texan with skin that turns just chocolaty enough to be exciting in the summer and an in-complete education. I kept flying a full schedule even after having my first child, as my husband went back to school and laboriously worked his way through his Master's degree. We lived in a travel trailer with books stuffed in all the storage compartments and hauled ourselves all the way from Texas to California. When the opportunity came to move to Waco for his PhD, the thought of being able to move back into a house delighted us so much that we put almost no thought into what life would be like in a small central Texas town.

Once in Waco and with renewed inspiration to resurrect some kind of a career for myself that would be more creative and keep me closer to home with my growing family, I visited a nearby saddle shop and bootmaker. The standard of workmanship was extraordinary and the boots particularly fascinated me. I tried my hardest to persuade the bootmaker to take me as an apprentice but had to settle for doing saddle shop repairs. My work bench was right next to the bootmaker's and for the next two years I became the annoying English lady behind the pile of old but repairable blankets full of horse shit, who never stopped asking questions.

During my time there, I made some of almost everything western, repaired all the English tack and mastered slicing yellow jackets out of the air with my shears. I also made my first pair of properly hand welted cowboy boots and several pairs of mules and shoes in my own time.

In order to progress with my career I began collecting the equipment I needed to make shoes and visiting any shoe or bootmaker who'd let me in their door. I bought my first industrial sewing machine and some leather, set up in my garage and made handbags. I sold the handbags in local stores and re-invested all the proceeds into more equipment, eventually buying an old run of shoe lasts, the all-important foot shaped molds that shoes are made on.

When I began making shoes for other people, I fully explained that it could take a while and a few re-makes till I get it right and I only charged them what it cost me to get the leather and other components. I quickly collected a list of willing customers all of whom had difficult shaped feet and had never found shoes that really fit. The bootmakers wise instructions on measurement and fit proved to be most thorough and I had little difficulty establishing a reputation of providing comfort. Making a women's shoe look sleek and modern without modern factory components is much harder than making them fit. It took a while before I gradually allowed customers to order top quality leather and more adventurous styles.

Manufactured women's shoes are beautiful and for the price there is little point in trying to make something prettier. The best and possibly the only good reason for buying hand-made shoes is comfort, superior materials and better fit, the latter of which is by far the majority of bespoke customers. Despite telling every single one of my customers to please come back for alterations if you are not completely comfortable and knowing that my instruction in old school construction was reliable, the persistent question of what foot ailments I should safely take on even under the instance of the most desperate customer, gnawed on me and I decided to become fully qualified as a pedorthist.

Since moving to Waco, I began running. No-longer living in the mountains or running from flight to flight it quickly became evident that just like everyone else in my age group I needed to do something to prevent myself from becoming a blob. I slogged it out on the stair-climber every morning until a svelte mom about my age bounced up to me and invited me to join her running group. My new coach ran circles back and forth between the varying levels of runners that she'd persuaded to join the class. As she herded us forward, we told stories and laughed till our sides split, before long and without realizing that I no-longer needed to walk intermittently, I became addicted.

I studied most of the pedorthic curriculum online, towards the end travelling to Tulsa, OK, to learn the practical side, fabricating orthotics and performing gait analysis. Just before my journey to Tulsa I had become interested in the minimal shoe trend and I listened to the audible version of *Born to Run* by Christopher Mc Dougal while driving. By the time I sat for my board exams to be a certified pedorthist I was completely immersed in my own research and learning project in the construction details and requirements of the minimal running shoe.

I had started running with the first generation of Vibram Five Fingers. They were far from fitting my skinny little feet so I sliced open the back and fudged a few adjustments to make them work. I soon developed 'top of the foot pain' which after a quick google search proved to be a remarkably common problem, I also stubbed my toe a few times and hobbled on in pain until resolving to find a better solution.

I went through countless prototypes in my studio, creating, adjusting, and then popping out for a quick run. The cost of materials and length of time to fabricate verses the speed in which I wore through the type of rubber soling available to me led me in the direction of buying cheap racing spikes, slicing the entire plastic sole off and replacing it with thin and flexible rubber. During the remodel of the first pair, I had one with the original 3mm foam lining and one that I had ripped the lining out, I put both on my feet and started standing on different soling products to see which one felt best. I inadvertently discovered that the 3mm foam gave me immediate knee pain and without it, not the tiniest twinge. Surprised and curious to understand why, I ran straight to the library, I cashed in on years of supporting my husband's academic career and enlisted his help to find studies and related papers.

Following the path of the dueling research papers from top scientists around the world is another addictive habit that seems at first like it would give you the answer although later reveals more questions that you now have to decide which would be more important to know the answer to first. It's been years now, I have a junk draw full of flash drives with info I might come back to at some stage and I still have more questions. Some of the more interesting subjects have led me into discussions with the authors and hopefully in the future I'll help design footwear solutions that solve some very real problems.

After running my way through several versions of my reconstructed running shoes, a British designer came out with Vivo barefoot running shoes, they were not quite how I would make them, but pretty good. I ran in them for the next year or two till Vapor gloves by Merrill came onto the market that I have worn ever since. There are a few things I would do differently if I were the designer, but for the most part they are pretty close to the ideal minimal running shoe.

Retrospectively the effects of minimal shoe running on my body have been most surprising. The first thing to be fixed, were my knees. With cushioned shoes I was a chronic runner's knee sufferer and never suffered a moment more from the day I went minimal. Except, one big crunch, less than a year in. A large bull dog leapt out and gave a huge bark from behind me, I stiffened with fear as I landed on my right leg turning in panic to look behind. My leg must have been too straight and I felt a big crunch. I was able to continue which is good because the dog turned out to be unaffected by mace or flying rocks and only retreated after a loose Chihuahua joined in the chase.

The next thing to change was strength verses pain. As I got stronger, my feet changed shape drawing up more in the arch and becoming denser. The added volume in my feet brought me welcome protection from the road and the tiny little pebbles that strike awkwardly into the thin soles. I think my feet truly stopped hurting after the first year. After the second year my form was noticeably better and my speed seemed more comparable to my shod counterparts. After the third year I no longer felt like my feet were at risk of overuse injury relative to the other parts of my body, and by year four I realized that previously I had had no idea what running was supposed to feel like.

Leather work is incredibly un-forgiving. One tiny miss-stitch makes a hole that is there forever and not only looks bad but undermines the integrity of the product letting in water and increasing the risk of a tear or early disintegration.

Back when I worked in the saddle shop I remember countless occasions of one or other of us just completely crushed at the loss of a piece we were working on due to what in other mediums would be ignored but in leather was considered devastation. The loss was always followed by an extensive apology to the owner. One time no one even knew my mistake, hours and hours into a project and buried under a pile of scraps too precious to be thrown away I gasped "SHIT" and, in the kind of a way that one might know of tragedy before a single word has been spoken, my call was answered with a chorus,

"Don't bleed on the leather!"

It was just a small cut and thankfully not a drop went on any of the leather.

Once working for myself the stress of mistakes only got worse. My margins were so tight that anything repeated meant making a loss for the month. I limited the quality of leather that I allowed my customers to order in attempt to minimalize my own anxiety. When finally I did begin ordering more extravagant leather and charging accordingly my shoes certainly became more beautiful with a luxurious feel that matched. Sadly the more I charged, the longer I took. I can't cut into a beautiful piece of calf or kangaroo if I'm not certain the pattern is perfect and then once I've got all my little pieces set, I carefully lower the sewing machine needle at the pace of a slow Sunday sermon.

Every tortured foot that I've carefully made shoes for and every hobbling person that I've helped stand a little taller has been an important learning experience. I will never become rich or even make more than a few bucks an hour making one lovely pair of shoes at a time and so for now I have to take a little break in making shoes for individual customers. I will return to it, not making shoes is like sending away a rebellious child, eventually you just have to open the door and let them back in.

As a shoemaker, everybody who walks in the door asks,

"What kind of shoes should I wear?" followed by,

"How do you know?"

The next thing they say is "My Doctor said I have that F*** thing.....and he has it too."

Next time I open my door for business I'll sell this little book to all who ask. The time saved in repeating these instructions, will probably still be spent in the intriguing perfectionism that keeps the honorable trade alive and relevant.

www.ingramcontent.com/pod-product-compliance
Lightning Source LLC
Chambersburg PA
CBHW070243290526
45789CB00004B/1741